Table of Contents

Understanding COPD: A Primer
    The Silent Threat: Understanding the Risks
    The Silent Symptoms: Recognizing the Signs of COPD
    Unmasking the Silent Thief: The Diagnostic Journey
    Unveiling the Treatment Plan: Managing COPD
    Breathing Easy: Managing Exacerbations
    Breathing Freely: The Power of Pulmonary Rehabilitation
    Navigating the World with COPD
    The Emotional Toll of COPD
    Empowering Yourself: Taking Control of Your COPD
    Breathing Easy: Tips for Daily Living with COPD
    Nourishing Your Body, Nourishing Your Lungs: The Role of Nutrition in COPD
    The Power of Exercise: A Breath of Fresh Air
    The Mind-Body Connection: Managing Stress and Anxiety
    The Role of Complementary Therapies in COPD Management
    Preparing for Emergencies: A Survival Guide for COPD Patients
    Advocating for Yourself: Taking Control of Your Healthcare
    Embracing a Positive Outlook: Living Well with COPD
    The Future of COPD Care: Hope on the Horizon
References

Understanding COPD: A Primer

What is COPD?

Chronic Obstructive Pulmonary Disease (COPD) is a progressive lung disease that makes it difficult to breathe. It's characterized by inflammation and narrowing of the airways, leading to airflow limitation. This condition primarily affects the lungs, but it can also impact the heart and other organs.

The Silent Thief of Breath

COPD not only affects the lungs but can also have a significant impact on other organs and systems. It can lead to:

- **Heart disease:** Increased risk of heart attacks, heart failure, and irregular heart rhythms.
- **Lung cancer:** A serious complication of COPD, particularly among smokers.
- **Osteoporosis:** Weakening of the bones, often linked to chronic inflammation.
- **Mental health issues:** Anxiety, depression, and sleep disorders can arise from the challenges of living with COPD.

The Toll of COPD

The impact of COPD on quality of life can be significant. Individuals with COPD may experience:

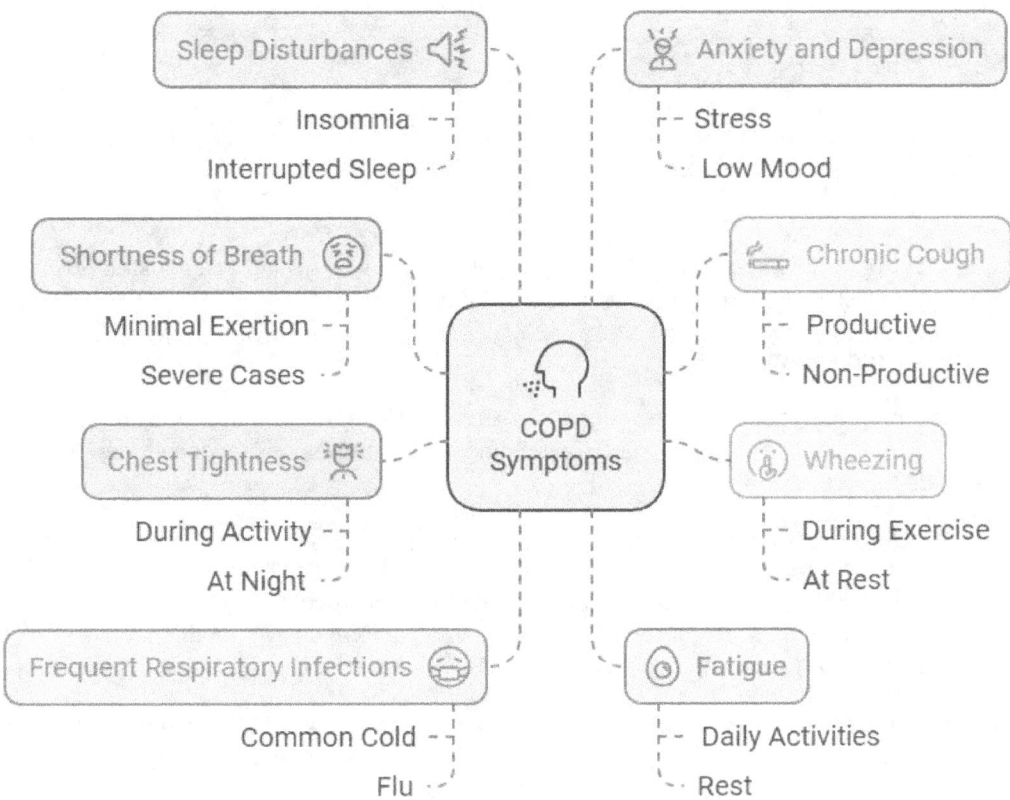

These symptoms can significantly impair daily activities, limit social interactions, and reduce overall well-being.

The Culprits Behind COPD

While the exact causes of COPD are complex and often multifaceted, several factors contribute to its development:

- **Smoking:** The most significant risk factor, particularly long-term smoking.
- **Exposure to irritants:** Chronic exposure to air pollutants, chemical fumes, and dust can damage the lungs.
- **Genetic factors:** Certain genetic predispositions can increase susceptibility to COPD.

- **Occupational exposures:** Certain occupations, such as mining and construction, involve exposure to harmful particles and fumes.

The Silent Progression

COPD is a progressive disease, meaning it worsens over time. As the lungs become increasingly damaged, symptoms may worsen, and individuals may experience more frequent and severe exacerbations.

A Glimpse into the Future

Understanding COPD is crucial for effective management. By recognizing the early signs and symptoms, seeking timely diagnosis, and adhering to a comprehensive treatment plan, individuals with COPD can improve their quality of life and slow the progression of the disease.

In the following chapters, we will delve deeper into the complexities of COPD, exploring various aspects of its management, including medical treatments, lifestyle modifications, and strategies for coping with the challenges of this chronic condition.

The Silent Threat: Understanding the Risks

While COPD can creep up on you, understanding the risk factors can help you take proactive steps to protect your lung health.

The Primary Culprit: Smoking

Smoking is the leading cause of COPD. The harmful chemicals in cigarette smoke damage the lungs, leading to inflammation and narrowing of the airways. The longer you smoke, the greater your risk of developing COPD.

The Role of Environmental Factors

Exposure to environmental pollutants can also contribute to the development of COPD. These pollutants include:

- **Air pollution:** Breathing in polluted air, especially from vehicle emissions and industrial activities, can damage lung tissue.
- **Occupational exposures:** Certain occupations, such as mining, construction, and farming, involve exposure to dust, fumes, and chemicals that can irritate the lungs.
- **Indoor air pollution:** Exposure to secondhand smoke, dust mites, mold, and pet dander can also contribute to lung damage.

Genetic Predisposition

In some cases, genetic factors can increase your susceptibility to COPD. A specific genetic disorder called alpha-1 antitrypsin deficiency can weaken the lungs and make them more vulnerable to damage.

Age and Gender

While COPD can affect people of all ages, the risk increases with age. Older adults are more likely to have been exposed to environmental pollutants and smoking for longer periods.

How to Reduce Your Risk

To minimize your risk of developing COPD, consider the following:

- **Quit smoking:** This is the single most important step you can take to protect your lung health.
- **Avoid exposure to irritants:** Limit exposure to air pollution, secondhand smoke, and other harmful substances.
- **Get regular check-ups:** Regular medical check-ups can help identify early signs of lung disease.
- **Practice good hygiene:** Wash your hands frequently to reduce the risk of respiratory infections.

- **Stay active:** Regular physical activity can help improve lung function.

By taking proactive steps to protect your lungs, you can reduce your risk of developing COPD and improve your overall health.

The Silent Symptoms: Recognizing the Signs of COPD

COPD often goes unnoticed in its early stages, as its symptoms can be subtle and easily mistaken for other conditions. Recognizing these early signs is crucial for early diagnosis and timely intervention.

The Stealthy Symptoms

Here are some common symptoms of COPD:

- **Chronic Cough:** A persistent cough that lasts for weeks or months, often producing mucus.
- **Shortness of Breath:** Initially noticeable during exertion, but progressing to shortness of breath even at rest.
- **Wheezing:** A whistling sound when breathing, particularly during exhalation.
- **Chest Tightness:** A feeling of pressure or constriction in the chest.
- **Frequent Respiratory Infections:** Increased susceptibility to colds, flu, and pneumonia.

The Silent Progression

As COPD progresses, symptoms may worsen, and individuals may experience:

- **Increased shortness of breath:** Difficulty performing daily activities, such as climbing stairs or carrying groceries.
- **Fatigue:** Chronic fatigue due to lack of oxygen.
- **Weight loss:** Unintentional weight loss, often due to decreased appetite and difficulty eating.
- **Anxiety and Depression:** The emotional toll of a chronic illness can lead to mental health issues.

The Silent Danger

COPD can lead to serious complications, including:

- **Respiratory Failure:** The lungs may not be able to provide enough oxygen to the body.
- **Pulmonary Heart Disease:** The heart may become overworked due to the increased effort required to pump blood through the lungs.
- **Increased Risk of Lung Cancer:** Smokers with COPD are at an increased risk of developing lung cancer.

- **Pneumonia:** People with COPD are more susceptible to pneumonia, a serious lung infection.

Breaking the Silence

If you experience persistent cough, shortness of breath, or other symptoms of COPD, it's important to seek medical attention. Early diagnosis and treatment can help slow the progression of the disease and improve quality of life.

By understanding the silent symptoms of COPD and taking proactive steps to address them, you can protect your lung health and live a fuller life.

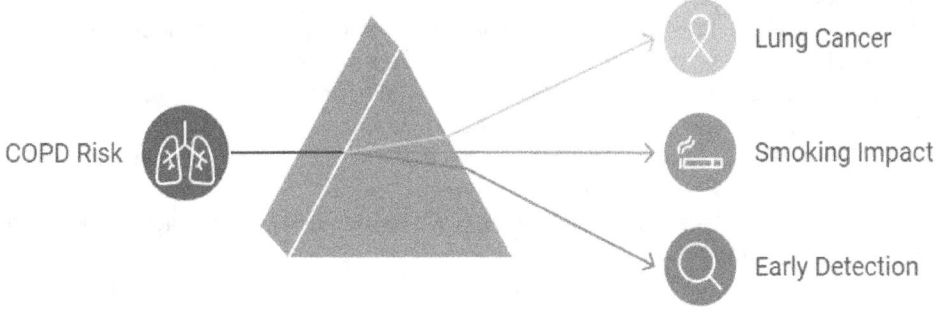

Unmasking the Silent Thief: The Diagnostic Journey

Once you've started noticing the subtle whispers of COPD, it's time to embark on a diagnostic journey. This journey isn't just about medical tests; it's about unraveling the mystery behind your symptoms and taking control of your health.

The Detective's Toolkit: Diagnostic Tests

Your healthcare provider is like a detective, using a variety of tools to uncover the clues that point to COPD. Here are some of the key tests they may use:

- **Pulmonary Function Tests (PFTs):** Imagine blowing into a tube as hard and as fast as you can. This simple act can reveal a lot about your lung function. PFTs measure how well your lungs work by assessing lung volume, airflow, and how efficiently oxygen and carbon dioxide are exchanged.
- **Chest X-ray:** A chest X-ray provides a snapshot of your lungs. It can help identify abnormalities like enlarged air sacs (emphysema) or thickened airways.
- **CT Scan:** A CT scan offers a more detailed view of your lungs. It can detect subtle changes in lung tissue, such as inflammation or scarring.
- **Blood Tests:** While blood tests won't directly diagnose COPD, they can help rule out other conditions and assess your overall health.
- **Pulse Oximetry:** This simple test measures the oxygen level in your blood. Low oxygen levels can be a sign of COPD.

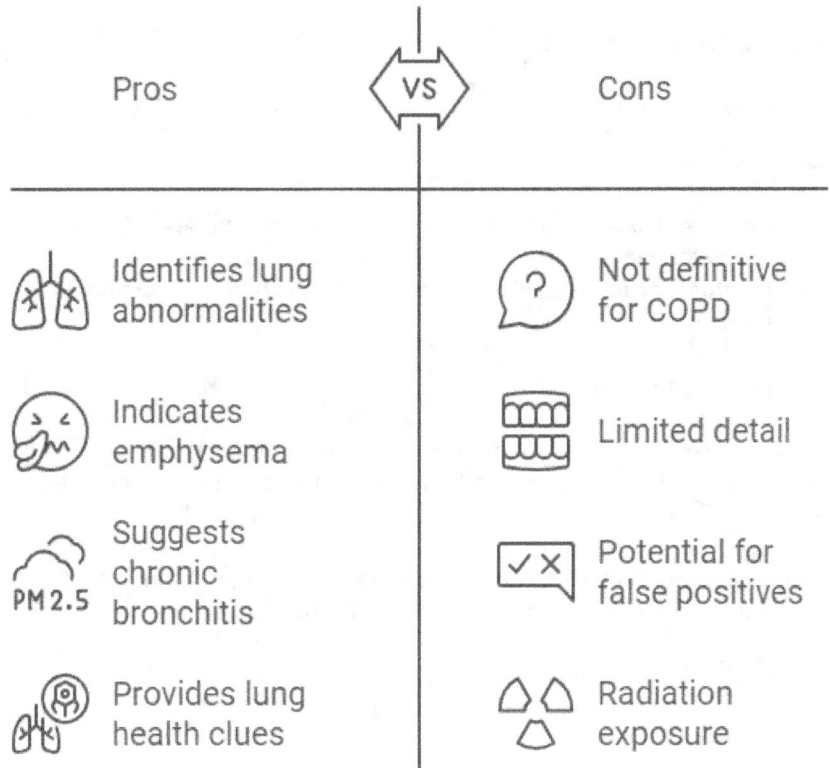

The Importance of Early Detection

Early diagnosis is crucial for effective management of COPD. By catching the disease in its early stages, you can take steps to slow its progression and improve your quality of life.

If you're experiencing persistent cough, shortness of breath, or other symptoms of COPD, don't delay in seeking medical attention. Remember, the sooner you address the issue, the better your chances of managing the disease and living a fulfilling life.

Unveiling the Treatment Plan: Managing COPD

Once a diagnosis of COPD has been confirmed, the focus shifts to developing a comprehensive treatment plan. This plan is tailored to your specific needs and aims to manage symptoms, improve lung function, and enhance your overall quality of life.

The Pillars of COPD Management

A typical COPD treatment plan involves a combination of strategies, including:

1. **Medications:**
    - **Bronchodilators:** These medications relax the muscles in the airways, making it easier to breathe.
    - **Inhaled Corticosteroids:** These medications reduce inflammation in the airways.
    -
    - **Combination Inhalers:** These inhalers combine bronchodilators and corticosteroids in one device for convenience.
2. **Pulmonary Rehabilitation:** This comprehensive program involves exercise training, education, and counseling. It helps improve lung function, muscle strength, and overall fitness.
3. **Oxygen Therapy:** For individuals with severe COPD, supplemental oxygen can help alleviate shortness of breath and improve quality of life.
4. **Lifestyle Modifications:** Making lifestyle changes, such as quitting smoking, eating a healthy diet, and engaging in regular physical activity, can significantly impact COPD management.

The Role of Lifestyle Changes

While medical treatments are essential, lifestyle modifications play a crucial role in managing COPD. Here are some key lifestyle changes to consider:

- **Quit Smoking:** Smoking is the leading cause of COPD, and quitting is the most important step you can take to improve your lung health.
- **Healthy Diet:** A balanced diet rich in fruits, vegetables, and whole grains can help reduce inflammation and boost your immune system.
- **Regular Exercise:** Engaging in regular physical activity, such as walking, swimming, or cycling, can improve lung function and overall fitness.
- **Stress Management:** Techniques like yoga, meditation, and deep breathing can help reduce stress and anxiety.

- **Avoid Exposure to Irritants:** Limit exposure to air pollution, secondhand smoke, and other irritants that can trigger COPD symptoms.

By combining medical treatments and lifestyle modifications, individuals with COPD can effectively manage their condition, improve their quality of life, and live a fulfilling life.

Breathing Easy: Managing Exacerbations

Exacerbations are periods of worsening COPD symptoms, often triggered by respiratory infections, air pollution, or other irritants. While they can be frightening, understanding how to manage them can help you maintain control of your condition.

Recognizing the Warning Signs

It's important to be aware of the signs of an impending exacerbation. These may include:

- Increased shortness of breath
- Increased cough
- Increased mucus production
- Change in mucus color (e.g., yellow or green)
- Wheezing
- Fatigue
- Fever

Taking Action: A Step-by-Step Approach

If you experience any of these symptoms, it's important to take immediate action:

1. **Follow Your Action Plan:** Your healthcare provider should have provided you with a personalized action plan, outlining specific steps to take during an exacerbation.
2. **Use Your Medications as Prescribed:** Adhere to your prescribed medication regimen, including both regular maintenance medications and medications for exacerbations.
3. **Stay Hydrated:** Drink plenty of fluids to help thin mucus and ease breathing.
4. **Rest:** Get plenty of rest to allow your body to recover.
5. **Avoid Irritants:** Stay away from smoke, air pollution, and other triggers.
6. **Seek Medical Attention:** If your symptoms worsen or don't improve, seek immediate medical attention.

Preventing Exacerbations

While it's not always possible to prevent exacerbations entirely, there are steps you can take to reduce your risk:

- **Get Vaccinated:** Stay up-to-date on flu and pneumonia vaccinations.
- **Practice Good Hand Hygiene:** Wash your hands frequently to reduce the risk of infection.
- **Manage Stress:** Stress can worsen COPD symptoms, so practice relaxation techniques like yoga, meditation, or deep breathing.
- **Avoid Exposure to Irritants:** Limit exposure to air pollution, secondhand smoke, and other irritants.

By recognizing the signs of an exacerbation, taking prompt action, and practicing preventive measures, you can minimize the impact of these events on your quality of life.

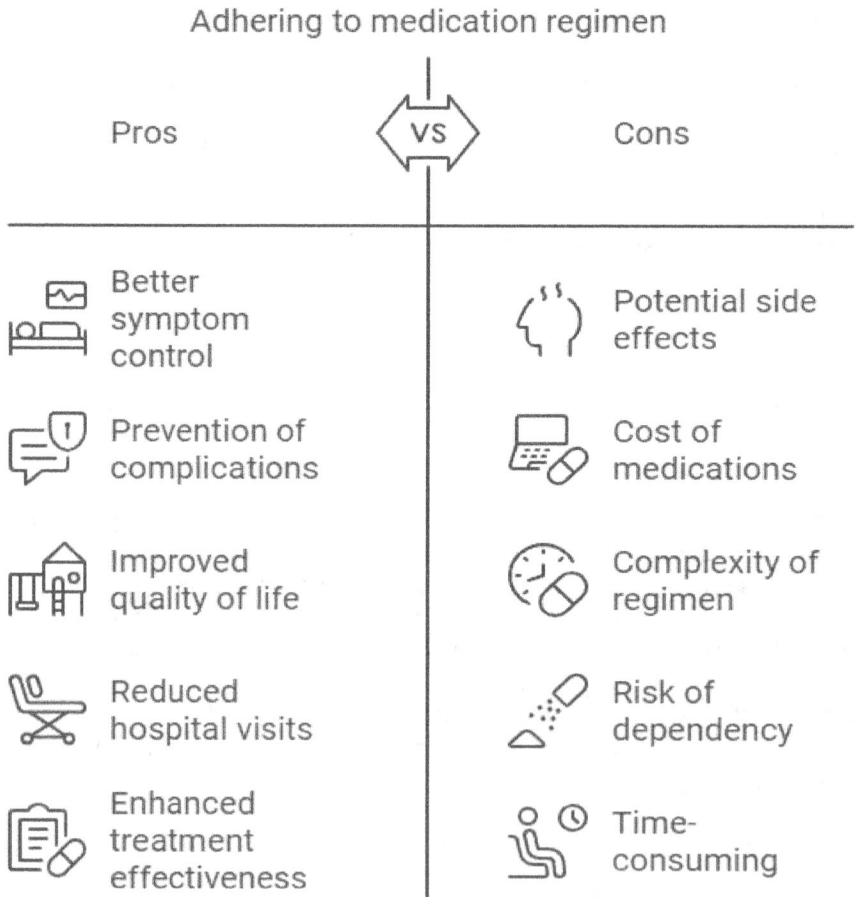

Breathing Freely: The Power of Pulmonary Rehabilitation

Pulmonary rehabilitation is a comprehensive program designed to help people with COPD manage their condition and improve their quality of life. This program involves a combination of exercise training, education, and counseling.

The Benefits of Pulmonary Rehabilitation

Pulmonary rehabilitation can help you:

- **Improve lung function:** Regular exercise can strengthen your respiratory muscles and improve your ability to breathe.
- **Reduce shortness of breath:** By improving your lung function and overall fitness, you can experience less shortness of breath during daily activities.
- **Increase energy levels:** Regular exercise can boost your energy levels and reduce fatigue.
- **Enhance quality of life:** By managing your symptoms and improving your overall health, you can enjoy a better quality of life.

What to Expect in Pulmonary Rehabilitation

A typical pulmonary rehabilitation program includes:

- **Exercise training:** Supervised exercise sessions tailored to your individual needs and abilities.
- **Education:** Learning about COPD, its management, and how to manage symptoms.
- **Counseling:** Addressing emotional and psychological issues related to living with a chronic illness.
- **Nutritional counseling:** Learning about the importance of a healthy diet in managing COPD.

Making the Most of Pulmonary Rehabilitation

To get the most out of your pulmonary rehabilitation program, it's important to:

- **Stay committed:** Attend all sessions and complete all exercises.
- **Ask questions:** Don't hesitate to ask your healthcare provider or therapist any questions you may have.
- **Practice what you learn:** Incorporate the techniques and strategies you learn into your daily life.
- **Stay positive:** A positive attitude can help you stay motivated and focused on your goals.

By participating in pulmonary rehabilitation, you can take control of your COPD and improve your overall well-being.

Navigating the World with COPD

Living with COPD doesn't mean you have to limit your lifestyle. With proper planning and preparation, you can continue to enjoy your favorite activities and travel the world.

Tips for Daily Living

- **Pace Yourself:** Break up tasks into smaller, manageable chunks.
- **Prioritize Activities:** Focus on essential tasks and delegate or postpone less important ones.
- **Use Energy-Saving Techniques:** Sit down to dress, use assistive devices, and avoid heavy lifting.
- **Manage Your Environment:** Keep your home clean and well-ventilated. Use air purifiers to improve indoor air quality.

Traveling with COPD

Traveling with COPD can be challenging, but it's not impossible. Here are some tips to help you plan your trips:

- **Consult Your Doctor:** Discuss your travel plans with your doctor to ensure you're healthy enough to travel.
- **Pack Essential Medications:** Bring a sufficient supply of your medications, including inhalers and oxygen, if needed.
- **Choose Your Destination Wisely:** Consider the climate and altitude of your destination.
- **Plan Ahead:** Research your destination and accommodations to ensure accessibility.
- **Pack Light:** Avoid carrying heavy luggage.
- **Stay Hydrated:** Drink plenty of fluids, especially during flights.

Coping with Exacerbations on the Go

If you experience an exacerbation while traveling, it's important to:

- **Rest:** Find a quiet place to rest and recover.
- **Use Your Medications:** Take your medications as prescribed.
- **Seek Medical Attention:** If your symptoms worsen, seek medical attention immediately.

Remember, with careful planning and preparation, you can continue to travel and enjoy life, even with COPD.

The Emotional Toll of COPD

Living with a chronic illness like COPD can take an emotional toll. It's common to experience a range of emotions, including frustration, anxiety, and depression.

Understanding the Emotional Impact

COPD can affect your emotional well-being in several ways:

- **Fear and Anxiety:** The uncertainty of the future and the fear of exacerbations can cause anxiety.
- **Depression:** Feeling overwhelmed by the challenges of COPD can lead to depression.
- **Social Isolation:** Difficulty breathing can limit social activities and lead to feelings of isolation.
- **Frustration:** Frustration with limitations and the inability to do things you used to enjoy.

Coping Strategies

Here are some strategies to help you cope with the emotional challenges of COPD:

- **Talk to Others:** Share your feelings with loved ones, friends, or a therapist.
- **Join a Support Group:** Connecting with others who understand what you're going through can be incredibly helpful.
- **Practice Relaxation Techniques:** Techniques like meditation, yoga, and deep breathing can help reduce stress and anxiety.
- **Set Realistic Goals:** Break down tasks into smaller, manageable steps.
- **Focus on the Positive:** Celebrate your achievements, no matter how small.
- **Seek Professional Help:** If you're struggling with depression or anxiety, consider seeking professional help.

Remember, it's okay to feel overwhelmed at times. By seeking support and practicing self-care, you can manage the emotional challenges of COPD and improve your overall well-being.

Empowering Yourself: Taking Control of Your COPD

Living with COPD doesn't have to define you. By taking an active role in your healthcare, you can empower yourself and improve your quality of life.

Building a Strong Partnership with Your Healthcare Team

A strong partnership with your healthcare team is essential for effective COPD management. Here are some tips for building a strong relationship with your healthcare provider:

- **Ask Questions:** Don't be afraid to ask questions about your condition, treatment options, and lifestyle changes.
- **Be Honest:** Be honest about your symptoms, concerns, and challenges.
- **Keep a Symptom Journal:** Track your symptoms, medications, and triggers to help you and your doctor identify patterns.
- **Stay Informed:** Stay up-to-date on the latest research and treatment options.
- **Advocate for Yourself:** Don't be afraid to advocate for your needs and ask for what you need.

Taking Charge of Your Health

Here are some tips for taking control of your COPD:

- **Adhere to Your Treatment Plan:** Take your medications as prescribed and attend all of your appointments.
- **Make Lifestyle Changes:** Quit smoking, eat a healthy diet, and exercise regularly.
- **Manage Stress:** Practice relaxation techniques like yoga, meditation, or deep breathing.
- **Get Enough Sleep:** Aim for 7-8 hours of sleep each night.
- **Join a Support Group:** Connecting with others who understand what you're going through can be incredibly helpful.
- **Stay Positive:** A positive attitude can help you cope with the challenges of COPD.

The Power of Hope

Living with COPD can be challenging, but it's important to maintain hope. By taking control of your health, you can improve your quality of life and live a fulfilling life.

Remember, you're not alone. There are many resources available to help you manage your COPD. With the right support and determination, you can overcome the challenges of this chronic condition and live a life you love.

Breathing Easy: Tips for Daily Living with COPD

Living with COPD can present daily challenges, but with the right strategies, you can manage your symptoms and live a fulfilling life. Here are some tips for navigating daily life with COPD:

Managing Daily Activities

- **Pace Yourself:** Break down tasks into smaller, manageable chunks.
- **Prioritize Activities:** Focus on essential tasks and delegate or postpone less important ones.
- **Use Energy-Saving Techniques:** Sit down to dress, use assistive devices, and avoid heavy lifting.
- **Plan Ahead:** Anticipate your needs and plan accordingly.

Creating a Healthy Home Environment

- **Good Ventilation:** Open windows and use fans to circulate air.
- **Regular Cleaning:** Dust, vacuum, and mop frequently to reduce allergens and irritants.
- **Avoid Irritants:** Reduce exposure to smoke, chemicals, and pet dander.
- **Consider an Air Purifier:** An air purifier can help filter out pollutants.

Traveling with COPD

Traveling with COPD can be challenging, but it's not impossible. Here are some tips:

- **Consult Your Doctor:** Discuss your travel plans with your doctor to ensure you're healthy enough to travel.
- **Pack Essential Medications:** Bring a sufficient supply of your medications.
- **Choose Your Destination Wisely:** Consider the climate and altitude of your destination.
- **Plan Ahead:** Research your destination and accommodations to ensure accessibility.
- **Pack Light:** Avoid carrying heavy luggage.
- **Stay Hydrated:** Drink plenty of fluids, especially during flights.

By implementing these strategies, you can make daily living with COPD more manageable and enjoyable.

Nourishing Your Body, Nourishing Your Lungs: The Role of Nutrition in COPD

A healthy diet plays a crucial role in managing COPD. By fueling your body with the right nutrients, you can improve your lung function, boost your immune system, and enhance your overall well-being.

Key Nutritional Considerations for People with COPD

- **Adequate Caloric Intake:** Maintaining a healthy weight is important for people with COPD. A balanced diet can provide the energy you need for daily activities.
- **Protein-Rich Foods:** Protein helps repair and build tissues, including lung tissue. Incorporate lean protein sources like chicken, fish, beans, and tofu into your meals.
- **Fruits and Vegetables:** These nutrient-packed foods are rich in antioxidants, which can help protect your lungs from damage.
- **Whole Grains:** Whole grains provide fiber, which aids in digestion and helps regulate blood sugar levels.
- **Healthy Fats:** Omega-3 fatty acids, found in fatty fish like salmon and flaxseed, can reduce inflammation.
- **Hydration:** Drinking plenty of fluids, especially water, helps thin mucus and keeps your airways moist.

Tips for Eating a COPD-Friendly Diet

- **Eat Smaller, More Frequent Meals:** This can help prevent indigestion and shortness of breath.
- **Choose Low-Sodium Foods:** Excess sodium can lead to fluid retention, which can worsen breathing difficulties.
- **Limit Alcohol and Caffeine:** Excessive alcohol and caffeine can dehydrate you and interfere with sleep.
- **Cook Smart:** Use cooking methods that minimize nutrient loss, such as steaming, grilling, and baking.

By making informed food choices and adopting healthy eating habits, you can support your lung health and improve your overall quality of life.

The Power of Exercise: A Breath of Fresh Air

Regular physical activity is a vital component of COPD management. It can help improve lung function, increase energy levels, and enhance your overall quality of life.

Benefits of Exercise for People with COPD

- **Improved lung function:** Regular exercise can strengthen your respiratory muscles, making it easier to breathe.
- **Increased energy levels:** Physical activity can boost your energy levels and reduce fatigue.
- **Enhanced quality of life:** Exercise can improve your mood, reduce stress, and improve your overall well-being.
- **Weight management:** Regular physical activity can help you maintain a healthy weight.

Types of Exercise for People with COPD

- **Aerobic exercise:** Activities like walking, swimming, and cycling can help improve lung function and cardiovascular health.
- **Strength training:** Building muscle strength can help with everyday tasks and improve your overall physical function.
- **Pulmonary rehabilitation:** A supervised exercise program that can help you improve your lung function and quality of life.

Tips for Exercising with COPD

- **Start slowly and gradually increase the intensity and duration of your workouts.**
- **Listen to your body:** If you experience shortness of breath or chest pain, stop and rest.
- **Choose low-impact activities:** Activities like swimming and water aerobics are gentle on your joints.
- **Exercise with a friend or family member:** Having a workout buddy can help you stay motivated.

By incorporating regular physical activity into your routine, you can take control of your COPD and live a more active and fulfilling life.

The Mind-Body Connection: Managing Stress and Anxiety

Living with a chronic illness like COPD can be stressful and anxiety-provoking. However, managing stress is crucial for your overall well-being.

The Impact of Stress on COPD

Stress can exacerbate COPD symptoms, such as shortness of breath, cough, and chest tightness. It can also weaken your immune system, making you more susceptible to respiratory infections.

Effective Stress Management Techniques

Here are some techniques to help you manage stress and anxiety:

- **Deep Breathing Exercises:** Deep breathing can help calm your mind and slow your heart rate.
- **Meditation and Mindfulness:** Mindfulness practices can help you stay present and reduce stress.
- **Yoga and Tai Chi:** These gentle exercises can improve flexibility, reduce stress, and enhance your overall well-being.
- **Progressive Muscle Relaxation:** This technique involves tensing and relaxing different muscle groups to promote relaxation.
-
- **Limit Caffeine and Alcohol:** Excessive caffeine and alcohol can worsen anxiety and sleep disturbances.
- **Get Enough Sleep:** Aim for 7-8 hours of quality sleep each night.
- **Connect with Others:** Spending time with loved ones can help boost your mood and reduce stress.

Seeking Professional Help

If you're struggling with severe anxiety or depression, consider seeking professional help from a mental health professional. Therapy and medication can help you manage your symptoms and improve your quality of life.

By incorporating stress management techniques into your daily routine, you can reduce the impact of stress on your mental and physical health.

The Role of Complementary Therapies in COPD Management

Complementary therapies can be used to complement traditional medical treatments for COPD. These therapies can help manage symptoms, improve quality of life, and reduce stress. However, it's important to consult with your healthcare provider before trying any new therapy.

Popular Complementary Therapies for COPD

- **Acupuncture:** This involves inserting thin needles into specific points on the body to stimulate the body's natural healing abilities. Acupuncture may help to relieve pain, reduce inflammation, and improve lung function.
-
- **Meditation and Mindfulness:** These practices can help reduce stress, anxiety, and depression, which can worsen COPD symptoms.
- **Yoga and Tai Chi:** These gentle exercises can improve flexibility, strength, and balance, as well as reduce stress and anxiety.
- **Massage Therapy:** Massage can help relax muscles, reduce pain, and improve sleep.
- **Herbal Remedies:** Some herbal remedies, such as ginger and licorice, may help to relieve cough and reduce inflammation. However, it's important to use herbal remedies with caution and consult with a healthcare provider.

Important Considerations

- **Consult Your Doctor:** Always consult with your healthcare provider before starting any new complementary therapy, especially if you are taking medications.
- **Choose Reputable Practitioners:** Ensure that you choose qualified and experienced practitioners.
- **Don't Replace Traditional Treatment:** Complementary therapies should not replace traditional medical treatments.

By incorporating complementary therapies into your COPD management plan, you may experience additional benefits and improve your overall well-being.

Preparing for Emergencies: A Survival Guide for COPD Patients

While it's important to maintain a positive outlook, it's also essential to be prepared for emergencies. By having a plan in place, you can minimize the impact of an exacerbation and ensure prompt medical attention.

Creating an Emergency Plan

- **Identify Your Triggers:** Understand what triggers your symptoms, such as air pollution, smoke, or cold weather.
- **Keep Essential Medications on Hand:** Ensure you have a sufficient supply of your medications, including inhalers, oral medications, and oxygen.
- **Know Your Emergency Contacts:** Keep a list of emergency contacts, including your doctor, emergency services, and a trusted friend or family member.
- **Develop an Evacuation Plan:** If you live in an area prone to natural disasters, have a plan for evacuating your home.
- **Prepare an Emergency Kit:** Assemble a kit with essential items, such as water, non-perishable food, a flashlight, and a first-aid kit.

Responding to an Exacerbation

If you experience a worsening of your COPD symptoms, follow these steps:

1. **Stay Calm:** Panicking can worsen symptoms.
2. **Use Your Medications:** Take your prescribed medications as directed.
3. **Rest:** Find a quiet place to rest and conserve energy.
4. **Hydrate:** Drink plenty of fluids to help thin mucus.
5. **Seek Medical Attention:** If your symptoms worsen or don't improve, seek immediate medical attention.

By being prepared for emergencies, you can minimize the impact of an exacerbation and ensure that you receive timely medical care.

Advocating for Yourself: Taking Control of Your Healthcare

As a person with COPD, it's important to advocate for yourself and ensure that you're receiving the best possible care. By being an active participant in your healthcare, you can improve your quality of life.

Tips for Effective Self-Advocacy

- **Educate Yourself:** Learn as much as you can about COPD, its symptoms, and treatment options.
- **Communicate Effectively:** Clearly communicate your symptoms, concerns, and goals with your healthcare provider.
- **Ask Questions:** Don't be afraid to ask questions about your diagnosis, treatment plan, and prognosis.
- **Seek Second Opinions:** If you're unsure about a diagnosis or treatment plan, consider seeking a second opinion.
- **Join a Support Group:** Connecting with other people who have COPD can provide emotional support and practical advice.
- **Keep a Symptom Journal:** Track your symptoms, medications, and triggers to help you and your doctor identify patterns.
- **Be Persistent:** If you're not satisfied with your care, be persistent and advocate for yourself.

Building a Strong Relationship with Your Healthcare Provider

- **Choose a Doctor Who Listens:** Find a doctor who is willing to listen to your concerns and answer your questions.
- **Be Prepared for Appointments:** Bring a list of questions and concerns to your appointments.
- **Be Honest:** Don't be afraid to share your honest feelings and experiences.
- **Trust Your Instincts:** If something doesn't feel right, don't be afraid to seek a second opinion.

By advocating for yourself, you can take control of your health and improve your quality of life.

Embracing a Positive Outlook: Living Well with COPD

Living with a chronic illness like COPD can be challenging, but it's important to maintain a positive outlook. By focusing on the positive and practicing self-care, you can improve your quality of life.

Cultivating a Positive Mindset

- **Practice Gratitude:** Focus on the things you're grateful for, big and small.
- **Set Realistic Goals:** Break down larger goals into smaller, achievable steps.
- **Celebrate Your Achievements:** No matter how small, celebrate your successes.
- **Practice Mindfulness:** Focus on the present moment and let go of worries about the future.
- **Connect with Others:** Spend time with loved ones and join a support group.
- **Seek Professional Help:** If you're struggling with negative emotions, consider talking to a therapist or counselor.

Self-Care Tips for COPD Patients

- **Prioritize Sleep:** Aim for 7-8 hours of quality sleep each night.
- **Manage Stress:** Practice relaxation techniques like yoga, meditation, or deep breathing.
- **Eat a Healthy Diet:** A balanced diet can help improve your overall health.
- **Exercise Regularly:** Engage in regular physical activity, such as walking, swimming, or cycling.
- **Avoid Triggers:** Identify and avoid triggers that worsen your symptoms.
- **Practice Good Hygiene:** Wash your hands frequently to reduce the risk of infection.

By adopting a positive mindset and practicing self-care, you can improve your quality of life and live well with COPD.

The Future of COPD Care: Hope on the Horizon

While COPD is a chronic condition, there is hope for the future. Ongoing research and advancements in medical technology are leading to new treatments and therapies that can improve the lives of people with COPD.

Emerging Treatments and Therapies

- **Novel Medications:** Researchers are developing new medications that target specific aspects of COPD, such as inflammation and mucus production.
- **Gene Therapy:** Gene therapy has the potential to repair damaged lung tissue.
- **Stem Cell Therapy:** Stem cell therapy may be used to regenerate lung tissue.
- **Pulmonary Rehabilitation:** Advances in pulmonary rehabilitation programs are leading to more effective treatments.

The Role of Technology

Technology is playing an increasingly important role in COPD management. Wearable devices can monitor lung function, heart rate, and oxygen levels, allowing patients to track their symptoms and make informed decisions about their health. Telehealth services can provide remote monitoring and support, making it easier for patients to access care.

Key Takeaways:

- **Understand Your Condition:** Knowledge is power. Educate yourself about COPD, its causes, symptoms, and treatment options.
- **Prioritize Lifestyle Changes:** Quit smoking, eat a healthy diet, and exercise regularly to improve lung function.
- **Seek Medical Care:** Regular check-ups and timely treatment are crucial for managing COPD.
- **Manage Stress:** Practice relaxation techniques like yoga, meditation, and deep breathing.
- **Connect with Others:** Join a support group or online community to share experiences and gain support.
- **Stay Positive:** A positive outlook can significantly impact your overall well-being.
- **Embrace Technology:** Utilize wearable devices and telehealth services to monitor your health.

Living with COPD can be a challenging journey, but it's important to remember that you're not alone. With the right knowledge, support, and medical care, you can manage your condition and live a fulfilling life. health and connect with healthcare providers. The future of COPD care is promising. Ongoing research and advancements in medical technology are leading to new treatments and therapies. By staying informed and actively participating in your healthcare, you can take control of your condition and live a fulfilling life.

Remember, every breath counts. Cherish each moment, and let hope be your guide.

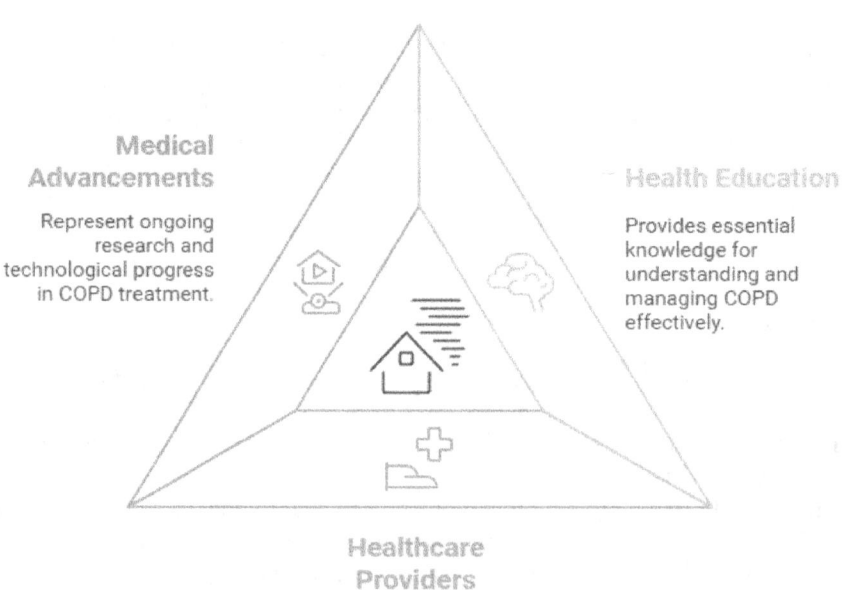

References

Global Initiative for Chronic Obstructive Lung Disease (GOLD). (2023). Global Strategy for the Diagnosis, Management, and Prevention of COPD, 2023 Report.

Hansel, N., & Pauwels, R. A. (2010). Severe chronic obstructive pulmonary disease. *The Lancet*, 376(9745), 1170-1180.

Rabe, K. F., Hurd, S. S., Anzueto, A., Barnes, P. J., Buist, A. S., Calverley, P. M. A., ... & Vogelmeier, C. F. (2007). Global strategy for the diagnosis, management, and prevention of chronic obstructive pulmonary disease: GOLD executive summary. *American Journal of Respiratory and Critical Care Medicine*, 176(6), 599-650.

Vestbo, J., Hurd, S. S., Agusti, A., Anzueto, A., Barnes, P. J., Fabbri, L. M., ... & Vogelmeier, C. F. (2013). Global strategy for the diagnosis, management, and prevention of chronic obstructive pulmonary disease: GOLD executive summary. *European Respiratory Journal*, 41(2), 255-296.

Singh, D., & Aggarwal, A. (2016). COPD exacerbations: Epidemiology, risk factors, and management strategies. *International Journal of Chronic Obstructive Pulmonary Disease*, 11, 1305-1317.

Agusti, A., & MacNee, W. (2013). Chronic obstructive pulmonary disease. *The Lancet*, 381(9873), 1343-1354.

Celli, B. R., & Martinez, F. J. (2015). Systemic effects of chronic obstructive pulmonary disease. *American Journal of Respiratory and Critical Care Medicine*, 192(1), 32-40.

Pauwels, R. A., Rabe, K. F., Buist, A. S., Calverley, P. M. A., Jenkins, C. R., & Hurd, S. S. (2001). Global strategy for the diagnosis, management, and prevention of chronic obstructive pulmonary disease: GOLD executive summary. *American Journal of Respiratory and Critical Care Medicine*, 163(5), 1256-1276.

Soriano, J. B., Soler, N., & Tordera, C. (2016). Non-pharmacological interventions for COPD: A systematic review and meta-analysis. *Respiratory Medicine*, 117, 1-10.

Sin, D. D., Bourbeau, J., Rabe, K. F., Anzueto, A., Barnes, P. J., Burkhart, D., ... & Vogelmeier, C. F. (2017). Global strategy for the diagnosis, management, and prevention of COPD, GOLD 2017 report. *European Respiratory Journal*, 50(1).

Tashkin, D. P., Celli, B. R., Sorkness, C. A., Burkhart, D., Kanner, R. E., & Make, B. (2007). A 12-month randomized trial of tiotropium vs salmeterol in COPD. *New England Journal of Medicine*, 356(22), 2220-2231.

Calverley, P. M. A., Vogelmeier, C. F., Barnes, P. J., Anzueto, A., Burkhart, D., Dekhuijzen, R., ... & Sin, D. D. (2017). Global strategy for the diagnosis, management, and prevention of COPD, GOLD 2017 report. *European Respiratory Journal*, 50(1).

Anzueto, A., Vogelmeier, C. F., Burkhart, D., Celli, B. R., Dekhuijzen, R., Fabbri, L. M., ... & Sin, D. D. (2017). Global strategy for the diagnosis, management, and prevention of COPD, GOLD 2017 report. *European Respiratory Journal*, 50(1).

Barnes, P. J., & Donnelly, L. E. (2010). New drugs for chronic obstructive pulmonary disease. *The Lancet*, 376(9745), 1181-1191.

Martinez, F. J., & Celli, B. R. (2009). Systemic manifestations and comorbidities of COPD. *Chest*, 136(3), 825-835.

Tal-Singer, R., & Kanner, R. E. (2010). Nutrition in COPD. *Chest*, 137(3), 956-964.
Goh, N. K., & Lim, T. K. (2012). Exercise training for COPD. *Respirology*, 17(5), 636-644.

Barnes, P. J. (2008). New drugs for COPD. *The Lancet*, 372(9640), 733-744.

Anzueto, A., Celli, B. R., Burkhart, D., Dekhuijzen, R., Fabbri, L. M., Martinez, F. J., ... & Sin, D. D. (2017). Global strategy for the diagnosis, management, and prevention of COPD, GOLD 2017 report. *European Respiratory Journal*, 50(1).

Calverley, P. M. A., Vogelmeier, C. F., Barnes, P. J., Anzueto, A., Burkhart, D., Dekhuijzen, R., ... & Sin, D. D. (2017). Global strategy for the diagnosis, management, and prevention of COPD, GOLD 2017 report. *European Respiratory Journal*, 50(1).

www.ingramcontent.com/pod-product-compliance
Lightning Source LLC
Chambersburg PA
CBHW030041230526
45472CB00002B/616